How I Treated My RA

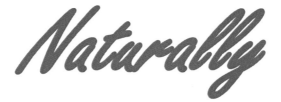

Naturally

Written by someone who chose a different path for her rheumatoid arthritis.

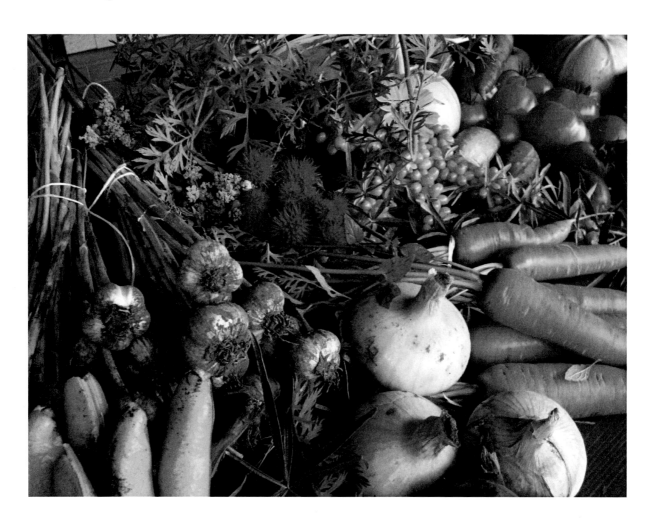

Sylvia Fulmer

TheHealthyFoodMaven

"The modern-day medical system will not train or permit the medical doctor (the MD) to address and conquer Autoimmunity (the root cause), responsible for over 100 autoimmune conditions including Rheumatoid Arthritis. The doctors are permitted to treat symptoms only. The root-cause, Autoimmunity, has become the "Protected Golden Goose" of the industry responsible for 85% of the revenue collected by the medical/pharmaceutical complex in total." *Dr. Ronald P. Drucker*

My Story

I was athletic and healthy as a horse growing up. I started taking piano and ballet when I was four. I was on the gymnastics and swim teams all through school, and went horseback riding every Sunday afternoon. I grew up in Pasadena, CA and every Saturday afternoon I would go with my dad to do grocery shopping. Back then meat was purchased at the butcher shop and freshly caught fish was purchased at the fish monger's. Produce was purchased at the store, gathered from your garden or picked from fruit trees in your yard or a neighbor's. There was no fear of GMO's, animals weren't shot up with antibiotics and hormones, and fish weren't "farm raised." I rarely got to eat junk food and fast food was permitted as an occasional treat. I didn't drink soda.

Then I went to college and entered the work force and the rest is diet demise history. It didn't happen all at once, but by the time I hit my thirties, my diet was shot. I was still very active so my weight wasn't a problem. I was rarely ill so I thought everything was fine. What I didn't realize was that inside, where I couldn't see, things were happening in my body. It wasn't until about eight years ago that I started to notice some changes. They were subtle and I hardly noticed, yet they subconsciously nagged at me.

I started noticing that I was having trouble standing for a long period of time. I was a choral music director and teacher, and found myself often pulling up a stool to sit on. Walking a distance was also becoming a problem. The library was seven blocks from where I lived. It used to be an easy walk. Now it was not so easy. I had to bring a stool into the kitchen if I was going to do a lot of cooking or baking because standing the whole time was out of the question. The pain in my back and fatigue became intense. Then came the day when I realized that I could no longer run. That was scary.

Because I was out of work with no insurance, it would be five years later that I would be able to see a doctor. During that time, my mobility decreased at an alarming rate. My new primary physician referred me to a pain doctor in Riverside, CA. I thought I had come for my back pain, but what the doctor discovered during my visit was that my lack of mobility was coming from my right hip, not my back. After several x-rays, an MRI and blood work, I was diagnosed with Rheumatoid Arthritis and Osteoarthritis. The Osteoarthritis had completely destroyed my right hip joint. In my shock my only thought was "I won't take those drugs." I knew people who had RA and I knew about the horrible drugs that were prescribed to treat it. I knew I didn't want them. When I got home, I went straight to my computer and started researching natural alternative treatments and nutrition.

I learned about the damage my poor eating habits had done. I read about the foods that cause inflammation in the body and inflammation causes pain. Before I started, I would cry myself to sleep every night because of the pain. I went cold-turkey and eliminated everything – dairy, wheat, gluten, meat, SUGAR. I eventually added a few things back like eggs. In less than a week I finally slept through the night. I lost my craving for sugar, and the pounds started dropping off effortlessly. I had energy.

It hasn't been easy. Completely changing how and what you eat is a challenge. But, I no longer miss the foods I thought I couldn't live without. I use coconut oil almost exclusively for cooking. I drink almond or coconut milk. I use organic sugars. There is a healthy and tasty substitution for everything. When I eat beef, it's only grass-fed and fish is only wild-caught-*never* farm raised. I buy organic. I eat raw vegetables as much as possible and fresh in-season fruit. It's all been so worth it.

This past October I had hip replacement surgery on my right hip. After every test in the book, my rheumatologist said the results showed no symptoms of autoimmune disease.

 I created a group on Facebook, Treating Rheumatoid Arthritis Naturally, which currently has over 200 members.

What Exactly Is Rheumatoid Arthritis?

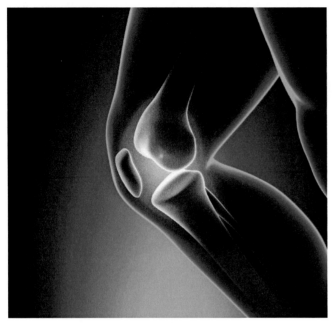

Rheumatoid arthritis (RA) is an autoimmune disease in which the body's immune system – which normally protects its health by attacking foreign substances like bacteria and viruses – instead attacks itself affecting the joints. This attack creates inflammation. If this inflammation goes unchecked, it can damage cartilage, as well as the elastic tissue that covers the ends of bones in a joint, and the bones themselves.

After a while there is loss of cartilage, and the joint spacing between bones can become smaller. Joints can become loose, unstable and painful, and lose their mobility. Joints can become deformed.

Rheumatoid diseases affect not only the joints and musculature but also the entire human organism and the patient's sense of well-being. A common misunderstanding among the public is that autoimmune disorders, such as RA, are merely joint discomforts when in fact rheumatoid and other autoimmune diseases are often an agonizing road that can lead to a premature death.

The cause of RA is not yet fully understood. About 1.5 million people in the United States have RA. Nearly three times as many women have the disease as men. In women, RA most commonly begins between ages 30 and 60. In men, it often occurs later in life. Having a family member with RA increases the odds of having RA; however, the majority of people with RA have no family history of the disease.

While only temporary symptomatic relief can be found from drugs, the cornerstone of conventional medical treatment often comes at the price of damaging ones health with pharmaceutical side effects.

Conventional Treatment

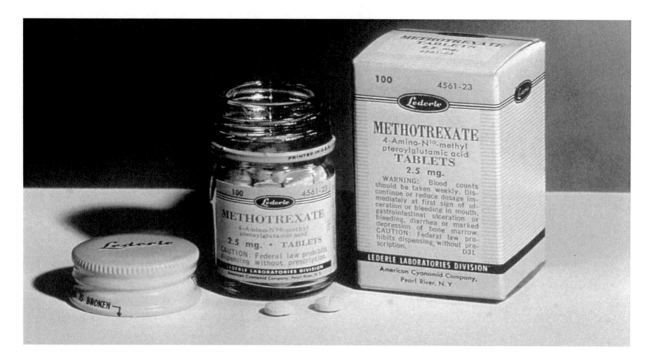

In terms of treatment, not much has changed in 2015. New drugs have been developed that carry with them even greater risks because most work by inhibiting the immune system. More alternative pills and therapies have arisen that still do not address causal factors. The reason for this may be found in a quote by Dr. Donald P. Drucker:

"The modern-day medical system will not train or permit the medical doctor (the MD) to address and conquer Autoimmunity (the root cause), responsible for over 100 autoimmune conditions including Rheumatoid Arthritis. The doctors are permitted to treat symptoms only. The root-cause, Autoimmunity, has become the "Protected Golden Goose" of the industry responsible for 85% of the revenue collected by the medical/pharmaceutical complex in total."

Drugs that are used will change over time. Traditionally prescribed drugs are steroids, whose side effects include severe osteoporosis, diabetes, mental instability, adrenal atrophy and progressive muscle wasting to Vioxx (Vioxx was taken off the market because of serious side effects) to Methotrexate (which was originally used for cancer and was noted for causing liver damage). Then there are the newer "'Biological Drugs" e.g. Enbrel, Remicaide and Humira. They work by disabling the immune system from performing its tasks. The risks from these drugs include tuberculosis, other infectious diseases and cancer. No drug cures and all drugs carry risks.

Whenever a new drug comes out the ads sing their praises – until the end of the commercial. Then they start telling the side-effects. When they're done, you feel like you're better off with whatever it is you have than take the drug. This is because conventional western medicine is about treating symptoms rather than addressing causes.

Healthy Eating and Its Effect on Chronic Inflammation and Joint Pain

We hear an awful lot about joint pain and chronic inflammation these days. It used to be only old people had sore joints. Now even young people are complaining. What's going on?

Normally inflammation is the body's defense system, but when it gets out of control, we have an overactive immune response and too much inflammation. Some of the results are allergies, rheumatoid arthritis, autoimmune disease, and asthma.

If chronic inflammation is left unchecked it can become a serious problem. What is not generally understood is that uncontrolled hidden inflammation the root cause of all chronic illness we experience.

Our joints are the structures that connect two or more bones in your body. Common joints are the hips, the knees, the hands, but there are many others as well. They are surrounded and cushioned by soft tissues. Joint swelling happens when fluid accumulates in these tissues. Pain, stiffness, or both may accompany the swelling as well. Often the joint will appear to be bigger than normal, or that its shape is somewhat irregular. Not all joint pain, however, is a symptom of a chronic condition, sometimes it can be a sign of an injury that requires medical attention.

One of the most frequent causes of joint swelling is arthritis. Osteoarthritis is the most common disorder of the joints, according to the United States National Center for Biotechnology Information (NCBI). Rheumatoid Arthritis is an inflammatory form of arthritis is also an autoimmune disease. While osteoarthritis occurs most often in older people, the onset of rheumatoid arthritis is usually between the ages of 25 and 50, but RA can appear at any age and can also be seen in children.

Conventional treatment for these conditions are anti-inflammatory drugs (ibuprofen or aspirin) and steroids such as prednisone. The problem is, while OK for treating acute problems, in chronic situations they tend to interfere with the body's own immune response and can lead to serious and sometimes deadly side effects.

The $64,000 question is, is there a better way of addressing the problem of inflammation? The answer is, yes.

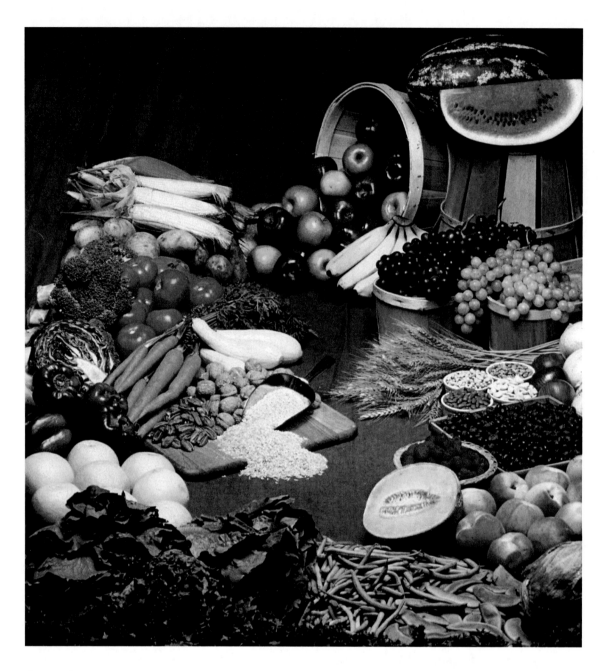

One of the most powerful tools to combat inflammation comes not from the pharmacy, but from the grocery store. Did you know that your diet can affect inflammatory responses within the body? It is well-known that the average American diet includes too *many* foods rich in omega-6 fatty acids found in processed and fast foods, and too *few* rich in omega-3 fatty acids such as those found in cold-water fish or supplements. Inflammation sets in when that balance is out of kilter.

Natural chemicals found in the plant foods-phytochemicals-are believed to help reduce inflammation. According to PMC, phytochemicals, which are natural compounds derived from fruits and vegetables, have shown anti-inflammatory and anti-cancer effects.

Foods that help fight inflammation:

- Animal-based omega-3 fat - wild-caught Alaskan salmon and fish or krill oil help fight inflammation throughout your body.
- Leafy greens - Dark leafy greens such as kale, spinach, collard greens and Swiss chard contain powerful antioxidants, flavonoids, carotenoids, and vitamin C. Opt for organic locally grown veggies that are in season, and consider eating a fair amount of them raw. Juicing is an excellent way to get more greens into your diet.
- Blueberries - Blueberries rate very high in antioxidant capacity compared to other fruits and vegetables. They are also lower in sugar than many other fruits.
- Tea - Tulsi aka Holy Basil is another tea loaded with anti-inflammatory antioxidants and other micronutrients that support immune function and heart health.
- Fermented vegetables and traditionally cultured foods - Optimizing your gut flora is important for a well-functioning immune system, and helps ward off chronic inflammation. In fact, the majority of inflammatory diseases start in your gut, as the result of an imbalanced microbiome. Fermented foods such as kefir, natto, kimchee, miso, tempeh, pickles, sauerkraut, olives, and other fermented vegetables, will help 'reseed' your gut with beneficial bacteria.
  Fermented foods can also help your body rid itself of harmful toxins such as heavy metals and pesticides that promote inflammation.
- Ginger - Studies have linked the root to a drop in joint pain caused by the chronic inflammatory conditions osteoarthritis and rheumatoid arthritis.
- Cherries - One fruit that stands out from the pack is the tart cherry. Like berries, the fleshy fruit abounds in anthocyanins (a type of phytonutrient), but it also delivers a uniquely powerful dose of anti-inflammatory compounds.
- Turmeric/Curcumin - Curcumin is the main active ingredient in turmeric. It has powerful anti-inflammatory effects and is a very strong antioxidant.

Foods to Avoid:

- Sugar - Foods high in sugar and saturated fat can spur inflammation. Learn all the different forms of sugar and *read the labels*!
- Dairy - Contrary to popular belief and advertisement, bone strength does not come from consuming milk and other dairy products but from plant foods. Dairy is a highly inflammatory food for most people. More processing ("skimming") does not make it any healthier, only more inflammatory.
- Grain-Fed Meat - Grain-fed animals that are kept in concentrated animal-feeding operations (CAFOs) are sick and unhealthy because they are not doing what comes naturally to them: grazing and living outdoors. They are barely kept alive by antibiotics, hormones, and other drugs. When we eat their meat, we become sick, too. And on top of it, processed meats are laced with preservatives, colorings, and artificial flavorings. Eat grass-fed only.
- Bad Fats - Vegetable oils (like corn, soy, and canola), all hydrogenated (or partially hydrogenated) oils, and all oils that have been heated for frying or deep-frying should be avoided. Coconut oil is the best.

- Agave - Despite its (questionable) reputation as a worry-free sweetener, agave is still full of sugar with a fructose content of up to 90 percent.
- Refined Carbohydrates - White flour products (breads, rolls, crackers) white rice, white potatoes (instant mashed potatoes, or French fries) and many cereals are refined carbohydrates. These high-glycemic index foods fuel the production of advanced glycation end (AGE) products that stimulate inflammation.
- Gluten and Casein - Common allergens like gluten and casein (proteins found in dairy and wheat) may also promote inflammation. For individuals living with arthritis who also have celiac disease (gluten allergy) and dairy intolerance, the inflammatory effect can be even worse. Gluten is found in wheat, rye, barley and any foods made with these grains. Casein is found in whey protein products.

Neither of these lists are exhaustive by any means, but they give you a place to start. Nutrition is the key. A miraculous thing, the immune system. It will defend the body against infectious organisms and other invaders, if we just give it what it needs - healthy food.

As much as possible, make sure you buy at least organic-preferably 100% certified organic.

Healthy Inflammation Fighting Foods

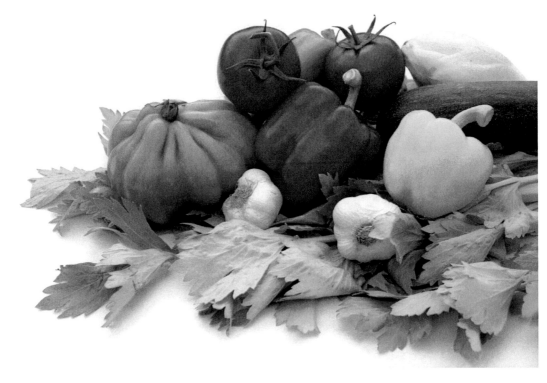

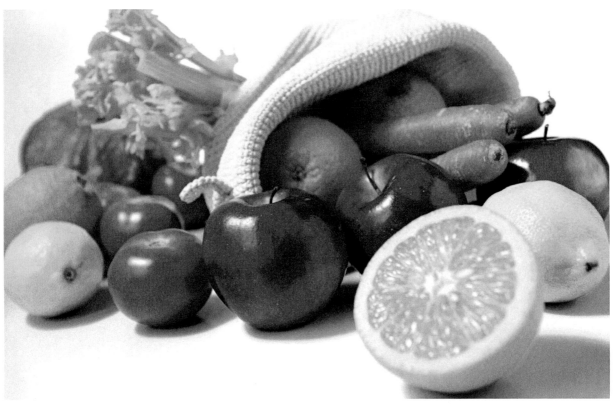

TURMERIC – *The Incredicle Miracle Herb*

Reduces side effects of chemotherapy

Aids in fat metabolism & weight management

Helps coughs

Strengthens ligaments

Skin tonic

Speeds up wound healing

Natural Analgesic

Natural antibiotic

Natural anti-inflammory

Blood purifier

Anti-arthritic

Improves digestion

Helps prevent gas/bloating

Helps prevent many cancers

Slows progression of MS

Prevents progression of Alzheimer's

Heals stomach ulcers

Improves skin conditions

Lowers cholesterol

Foods that FIGHT Inflammation

Broccoli	Cranberries	Oregano	Mulberries
Spinach	Pineapple	Parsley	Cocoa
Cauliflower	Cantaloupe	Rosemary	Hazelnuts
Cabbage	Brown Rice	Thyme	Avocado Oil
Green Beans	Turmeric	Barley	Basil
Sweet Potatoes	Walnuts	Kale	Anchovies
Ginger	Cloves	Cinnamon	Almonds
Salmon (wild)	Ground Flaxseed	Coconut Oil	Tuna
Papaya	Blueberries	Avocados	Chard
Collards Greens	Almond Butter	Red Beets	Radishes
Quinoa	Figs	Plums	Strawberries
Raspberries	Cherries	Kiwi	Pumpkin
Zucchini	Bell Peppers	Leeks	Rhubarb
Garlic	Lemons	Limes	Green Tea
Cucumber	Cilantro	Apples	Grapes
Mint	Red Cabbage	Olives	Asparagus
Cayenne Pepper	Jicama	Squash	Seaweed
Brussels Sprouts	Flaxseed Oil	Acai	EV Olive Oil

Foods that CAUSE Inflammation

Gluten

Casein

Oils
    Safflower
    Sunflower
    Soy
    Corn

Processed Meats
    Bologna
    Hot Dogs
    Ham
    Bacon
    Salami
    Lunch Meats
    Canned Meat

Fried Food

Meat & Dairy

Syrup & Soft Drinks

Fast Food

Packaged Food
    Mac n' Cheese
    Frozen Dinners
    Cake Mixes

Junk Food
    Potato Chips
    Candy
    Cookies
    Pudding
    Yogurt

Different Diets to Help Ease Rheumatoid Arthritis

There are foods that do help lower inflammation throughout your body, and what you put on your plate may help you manage your RA symptoms. Which diet is best for you? Decisions, decisions. If you ask your friends, *everyone* has an opinion.

A good place to start is with one of the world's oldest ways of eating, which has stood the test of time.

The traditional Mediterranean diet

Loaded with fruits, vegetables, whole grains, healthy fats, beans and fish, the traditional Mediterranean diet is probably as healthy as it gets. These foods have natural chemicals that keep inflammation in check.

Olive oil, another healthy fat, is a great alternative to take the place of full-fat dairy products like butter. That's good news for people with RA, because olive oil can lower the levels of the chemicals that cause inflammation.

The fruits and vegetables that are included in the diet are full of antioxidants. Antioxidants also help control inflammation. Deep or bright colors usually mean higher antioxidant levels. Think blueberries, blackberries, squash, sweet potatoes, carrots, tomatoes, peppers, oranges, broccoli, and melons.

For more information on The Mediterranean Diet go to bit.ly/1WXybG5.

Paleo diet

"The Paleo Diet is based upon everyday, modern foods that mimic the food groups of our pre-agricultural, hunter-gatherer ancestors. The following seven fundamental characteristics of hunter-gatherer diets will help to optimize your health, minimize your risk of chronic disease, and lose weight." Loren Cordain, PhD-Founder of the Paleo Movement

1. **Higher protein intake**
2. **Lower carbohydrate intake and lower glycemic index**
3. **Higher fiber intake**
4. **Moderate to higher fat intake dominated by monounsaturated and polyunsaturated fats with balanced Omega-3 and Omega-6 fats**
5. **Higher potassium and lower sodium intake**
6. **Net dietary alkaline load that balances dietary acid**
7. **Higher intake of, vitamins, minerals, antioxidants, and plant phytochemicals**

Here is a basic guide of what to eat on The Paleo Diet:

Eat

- Grass-produced meats
- Fish/seafood
- Fresh fruits and veggies
- Eggs
- Nuts and seeds
- Healthful oils (Olive, walnut, flaxseed, macadamia, avocado, coconut)

Don't Eat

- Cereal grains
- Legumes (including peanuts)
- Dairy
- Refined sugar
- Potatoes
- Processed foods
- Salt
- Refined vegetable oils

For more information on the Paleo diet go to bit.ly/**1KrhTAh**

GAPS diet

The beauty of the GAPS diet is that it is designed to be a temporary healing diet, with the promise that the majority of people heal within 3 years and can expand their diet again. It is basically no refined oils, refined sugars, dense starches, grains, or soy. Most legumes are restricted as well. Some raw dairy is allowed if tolerated.

The GAPS diet slowly heals the gut, strengthens the immune system. GAPS can help clear many health issues. Differing from a grain-free diet, GAPS removes all sugars (except a bit of raw honey), most dairy, most legumes and all disaccharides from the diet.

Rich in bone broths, vegetables, meats, healthy fats and fermented foods, GAPS is a therapeutic diet (usually followed for about one year) and not meant for the long-term or for those pregnant or nursing.

For more information on the GAPS diet go to bit.ly/1JC3ufl

Everyone is different and what works for one may not work for another. You may even find yourself taking some things from one diet and other things from another diet. What's important is that you find what works best for you. No one knows your body like you do.

You can also work out your own elimination diet. I just went cold turkey and quit everything-dairy, sugar, wheat, gluten, junk food, fast food, packaged food. Then I gradually added a few things back. I still don't do packaged food, junk food or fast food, sugar, and most dairy.

You'll know when you hit the right combination, your body will thank you.

Exercise

I know the last thing you want to hear is me telling you to move. You're already in pain and the thought of moving-as in exercise-is just repulsive. I'm here to tell you, exercise is really important. Getting plenty of exercise is an important part of coping with rheumatoid arthritis. It can help alleviate joint pain and stiffness, make you more flexible, improve your sleep, and boost your endurance.

Walking strengthens your bones and helps prevent osteoporosis. After menopause all women are prone to weaker bones, but it's more common among those who have RA and take steroids to treat inflammation.

If you already have RA, heart disease is another condition that you're more likely to get. Aerobic exercise, the kind that makes your heart pump faster, can help you control your weight thereby taking a lot of stress off your heart.

Here are some tips for success:

- Start slowly.
- Set a goal: Maybe you want to lose a few pounds, get in better shape for a trip, or walk a 5K.
- Once you have your big goal, set small targets along the way and chart your progress.
- Reward yourself when you meet each goal.

If you are not currently working out or exercising, you may also want to consult with a physical therapist to make a safe, effective workout plan.

Low-impact activities, like walking, swimming, bicycling, or using an elliptical machine are best. Any of these will get your heart pumping and classify as cardio or aerobic exercise.

Strength training uses resistance to work your muscles. You can use machines at a gym, hand-held weights, resistance bands, or even your own body weight. It strengthens muscles and increases the amount of activity you are able to do.

Stretching exercises are great but they should be gentle. Never, ever stretch a muscle that's not warmed up.

Be careful about activities that put a lot of stress on a joint, or are "high-impact," such as jogging, especially on paved roads, and heavy weight lifting. Try and do 20 to 30 minutes (or more) of low-impact conditioning exercise on as many days as you feel you can. Remember, some is better than none!

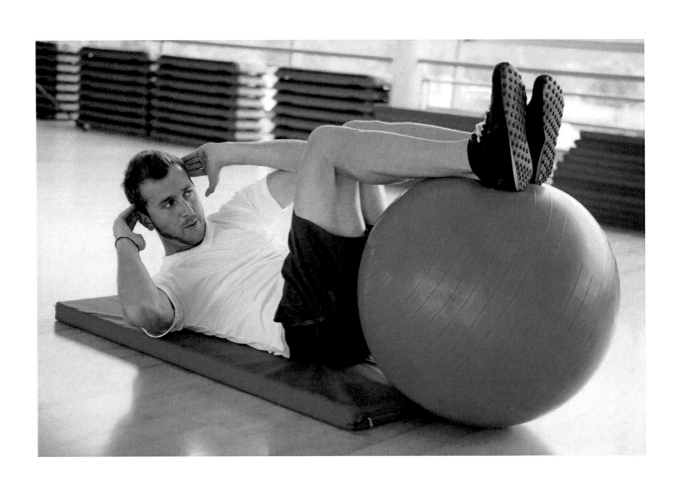

Hang In There!

The biggest part of being able to live with your RA is keeping a positive attitude. Unless they have experienced it, the average person is not going to be able to fully understand what you're going through. When you can get past their ignorance and shift your focus, you will find you actually feel much better than if you took them to task for their lack of knowledge about your condition. Why is that? Remember this equation: **STRESS=INFLAMMATION=PAIN**.

Research shows that when people have a chronic illness, there is a high risk of developing depression within two years of diagnosis. Maintaining a sense of humor in spite of all that's going on in your body can help keep you from sinking into depression.

"In an inflammatory type of arthritis such as RA, the pain caused by inflammation of the joints may come before depression, but then having depression may mean that the patient experiences his or her pain more severely than a patient with similar degrees of inflammation without depression," explains Angelica Gierut, MD, a rheumatologist and assistant professor of allergy, immunology, and rheumatology at Loyola University Medical Center in Maywood, Illinois.

Boosting your emotional health

At times you may feel hopeless or in despair because of your arthritis. Give your emotional health a boost, starting with these stress-busting recommendations:

- Relax - Even if it's only for 15 minutes.
- Breathe - Practice simple deep-breathing techniques.
- Exercise – Move, even in a limited way.
- Soak in a hot bath – Great for your pain, great for your spirits.
- Talk it out – Sometimes all you need to do is let your feelings out.
- Take a class inn emotional well-being – Can lead to a decrease in mental distress.

Although RA can be a challenging disease to live with, taking the right steps to boost your emotional health may help improve your physical pain as well.

Recipes

Can't let you get away without giving you a few recipes to start you out. Hope you enjoy them. Bon Appetite!

Amazing Anti-Inflammatory, Gut Healing, Blood Purifying Sleepytime Drink from *"Healthy Holistic Healing"*

Ingredients:

- 2 cups coconut milk (or milk of your choice)
- 1 teaspoon turmeric
- 1/4 teaspoon black pepper (the absorption of turmeric is actually **enhanced** when combined with black pepper)
- raw honey to sweeten, if desired

Directions:

- In a saucepan add all ingredients (except honey, if using) and whisk to combine
- Heat over medium heat until it starts to bubble
- Then turn heat down to low and simmer for about 5 minutes so the flavors meld
- Strain out the ginger
- Add honey and stir
- Makes 2 servings, so you can share the love

The Anti-inflammatory Smoothie from *"Food Babe"*

Ingredients:

3 tablespoons Nutiva hemp protein powder
2 inch piece of ginger (peeled if not organic)
2 cups of leafy greens (kale, collards, romaine, spinach, chard, etc.)
1 cup of celery
1 cup of mixed frozen berries of your choice (strawberries, blueberries, cranberries)
½ cup filtered water

Instructions:

1. Place all ingredients in a blender and blend for 1 min or until smooth
2. Serve immediately or store in airtight container for up to 1 day

Melt in Your Mouth Kale Salad from *"Food Babe"*

Ingredients

- 1 bunch of lacinato or dinosaur kale, stems removed, rinsed and patted dry
- ⅓ cup currants (or chopped raisins)
- juice of one lemon
- 1 tbsp of olive oil
- 1 tsp local honey
- ½ cup pine nuts toasted
- salt and pepper to taste
- 4 tbsp grated raw parmesan cheese

Instructions

1. In a food processor, process kale into small chopped pieces
2. To make dressing, stir lemon juice, olive oil, honey, salt and pepper together in a large bowl
3. Add chopped kale, currants, pine nuts and parmesan to bowl with dressing
4. Stir all ingredients together and serve
5. (Optional - Save some pine nuts and/or parmesan cheese for top of salad before serving for presentation purposes)

Thank You!

Thank you for taking the time to read this little book. I hope it is some help. The past two years have been a journey I never expected. I have met many people on this same journey. We can all learn from each other and encourage each other. Every day we learn more about RA. God made a miraculous immune system. It works very well when it is given what it needs – proper nutrition. It has worked for me and thousands of others. I hope you have equal success. God Bless You.

Follow me on Facebook:

"The Healthy Food Maven"

Join my Facebook group:

"Treating Rheumatoid Arthritis Naturally"

Follow me on Twitter:

"@hltyfdmaven"

Join my blog:

http://thehealthyfoodmaven.com

*Don't worry if it takes a couple of seconds to load.

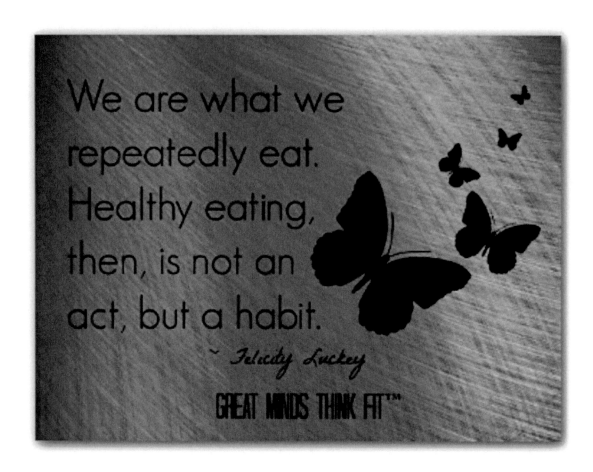

We are what we repeatedly eat. Healthy eating, then, is not an act, but a habit.

~ Felicity Luckey

GREAT MINDS THINK FIT™

THE END

29331879R00017

Made in the USA
Middletown, DE
15 February 2016